# THINK,
# LEARN,
# SUCCEED
## • WORKBOOK •

# THINK, LEARN, SUCCEED

## • WORKBOOK •

Understanding and Using Your Mind to
Thrive at School, the Workplace, and Life

# DR. CAROLINE LEAF

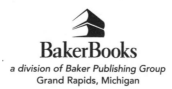

BakerBooks

*a division of Baker Publishing Group*
Grand Rapids, Michigan

Published by Baker Books
a division of Baker Publishing Group
P.O. Box 6287, Grand Rapids, MI 49516-6287
www.bakerbooks.com

Printed in the United States of America

ISBN: 978-0-8010-9355-5

Portions of this text taken from *Think, Learn, Succeed*, published by Baker Books, 2018

The Switch On Your Brain 5-Step Learning Process and The Metacog are registered trademarks of Dr. Caroline Leaf.

This publication is intended to provide helpful and informative material on the subjects addressed. Readers should consult their personal health professionals before adopting any of the suggestions in this book or drawing inferences from it. The author and publisher expressly disclaim responsibility for any adverse effects arising from the use or application of the information contained in this book.

20   21   22   23   24        7   6   5   4   3

In keeping with biblical principles of creation stewardship, Baker Publishing Group advocates the responsible use of our natural resources. As a member of the Green Press Initiative, our company uses recycled paper when possible. The text paper of this book is composed in part of post-consumer waste.

# Contents

Introduction   7

How to Use This Workbook   9

KEY 1: Are You Succeeding or Just Surviving?   11

KEY 2: The Mindset Guide, Part 1   17

KEY 3: The Mindset Guide, Part 2   29

KEY 4: The Gift Profile, Part 1   41

KEY 5: The Gift Profile, Part 2   49

KEY 6: The Switch On Your Brain 5-Step Learning Process, Part 1   59

KEY 7: The Switch On Your Brain 5-Step Learning Process, Part 2   67

KEY 8: The Science, Part 1   75

KEY 9: The Science, Part 2   85

Conclusion   94

# Introduction

What is success? What is learning? What is happiness? How do you create a life of meaning? How do you discover your purpose in life?

Regardless of what our society may say, success is not a matter of being like someone else or following some set pattern for your life. Success is all about *mental self-care*. Success goes beyond mindfulness into a lifestyle of cognitive transformation that is both sustainable and organic—and suited to who you are at your core.

Yet in a world that often defines success by your number of Instagram followers or number of digits in your income, it can be difficult to be successfully *you*. Indeed, with the fast pace of modern life and the overwhelming amount of information now at our fingertips, it is a challenge to take the time to think, learn, and succeed at life in your own wonderful way, which is why I decided to write my book *Think, Learn, Succeed: Understanding and Using Your Mind to Thrive at School, the Workplace, and Life.*

I wanted to show you that you are as successful as you want to be, in a unique way only you can be! You can use your unique way of thinking, feeling, and choosing to improve your overall intellect, cognitive performance, and mental and physical well-being. Harnessing these

7

natural resources will give you power over the present, depth and context to the past, and anticipation for the future.

I created this workbook as a guide to help you understand and apply the principles of deep, focused thinking and learning that lead to this type of success as discussed in *Think, Learn, Succeed*. Each key follows the main themes of the chapters in the book, with a series of questions that will help you understand and apply the information. Some questions may be repeated or asked in different ways—this is not an error! Repetition and the process of asking, answering, and discussing are integral to cognitive development; it is always important to ask a lot of questions from a variety of perspectives.

# How to Use This Workbook

This workbook is part of a three-part curriculum:

1. The *Think, Learn, Succeed* book
2. The *Think, Learn, Succeed* DVD
3. The *Think, Learn, Succeed* workbook

Both the DVD and workbook are organized around nine "keys" for a nine-week study. That is sixty-three days, although you can work through the study in more or less time if desired. It takes around twenty-one days to rewire neural pathways and begin building a new way of thinking about your life. It takes an additional forty-two days (two more sets of twenty-one days) for a total of sixty-three days to establish a new habit. Thus this workbook is designed to help you establish a habit of thinking and learning that will lay the foundation for a successful life.

As you work through each key, be as specific and honest as you can. Research shows change happens when we use our minds to develop our understanding. I would recommend working through the questions a second time after you have completed the workbook and as you use the Mindset Guide, the Gift Profile, and the 5-Step Learning

Process, which will help you better understand and apply the principles in *Think, Learn, Succeed*.

When you begin to follow the guidelines of *Think, Learn, Succeed*, your life will begin to change for the better. You will begin to understand how to learn effectively, change your circumstances, increase your creativity, improve your memory and its functionality, increase your emotional control, allow your emotions and stress to work for you and not against you, and experience intellectual satisfaction. You will realize that *you* are captain of your soul. You will recognize that no matter what your circumstances are, no matter what people tell you, and no matter what doubts you have had about yourself, you are designed to succeed. You will learn that you have the power to go from surviving to *thriving*!

# Are You Succeeding
# or Just Surviving?

Read pages 19–34 in *Think, Learn, Succeed* and watch the key 1 video.

1. *Today, most people can access vast amounts of information, yet few people know how to process this information and use it to be successful at school, work, and life.* How has this overload of information affected your life? Do you find it difficult to know what to think or believe? How do you use information to your own benefit?

_____

_____

_____

_____

_____

_____

_____

2. *We now have the world at our fingertips, yet, paradoxically, more and more of us live solitary, futile lives.* How has the technological revolution benefited you? How has it hindered you? How much time do you spend online? Has this impacted your social life?

_____

_____

_____

_____

_____

_____

_____

_____

_____

3. *When we gather information like puzzle pieces without putting the puzzle together, intellectual growth is stifled. This is a crisis of quantity over quality, and the consequences are frighteningly evident in society.* How do you make use of information? How do you think the overload of information, whether truth or "fake news," has impacted our society? How do you think our ability to think, learn, and concentrate has changed?

_____

_____

_____

_____

_____

_____

_____

_____

_____

4. *Rather than asking what is wrong with our society and the kind of thinking it promotes, we place the blame squarely on an individual's shoulders—or more to the point, their brain—divorcing him or her from the context of daily life.* How do labels such as "attention deficit" or "learning disabled" hinder people? Can such labels be beneficial? Does looking at what is wrong with an individual, rather than what is wrong with our society, change the way we view issues such as ADHD and loneliness?

_____

_____

_____

_____

_____

_____

5. *The point of thinking, learning, education, technology, medicine, and philosophy should be to build a better world, with connectedness and humanness as its core fundamental purpose.* Do you feel like this is true in your life? If yes, how? If no, why? What makes knowledge and learning significant? What makes work a vocation, or something with purpose? Why do we generally ask people what they do but not why they do it? How do we get from A, knowledge, to B, significance? How do you think that the technological revolution has helped us create a better world? How has the technological revolution hindered our progress as a species?

_____

_____

_____

_____

_____

_____

6. *We need to recognize that neither society nor our brains are the only factors in determining what we do with our lives.* How do our own choices impact our ability to think, learn, and succeed? Can we overcome our circumstances, or are we a victim of where, when, and how we live or what happens to us?

_____

_____

_____

_____

_____

_____

_____

_____

_____

_____

7. *Your ability to think, feel, and choose is innately powerful and resilient—you have a mind that is more potent than all the smart-phones on the planet combined!* Do you feel that this is true in your own life? If yes, how? If no, why? Do you think that it is possible to change your thinking, and, in turn, change your life?

_____

_____

_____

_____

_____

_____

_____

_____

_____

_____

8. *In recent years, in an attempt to address these modern challenges to thinking and learning, neuroscience has become very popular. It is almost as though adding the prefix "neuro," as in neuro-education, neuroleadership, neurospirituality, and so on, gives the method, course, program, or book more clout, thereby increasing its credibility.* Have you noticed this trend? How so? Is our current obsession with neuroscience helpful, or does it affect our ability to see beyond our biology?

_____

_____

_____

_____

_____

_____

_____

9. *Research has revealed that neuromyth beliefs are remarkably prevalent among the general public, educators, and even neuro-scientists (training in neuroscience does not necessarily translate to psychology or education!), hence the potential for interpretive errors to creep in, doing more harm than good.* What are these "neuromyths"? How do they impact our ability to think, learn, and succeed? Why do they represent a "reductionistic" mentality? Can you think of examples of "neuromyths" in your life?

_____

_____

_____

_____

_____

_____

_____

10. *Science, of course, advances through trial and error.* How does science advance? How can science be misused or misunderstood? How does this relate to the above mentioned "neuromyths"?

_____

_____

_____

_____

_____

_____

11. *Regardless of what anyone has told you, you can learn.* Has what other people have told you about your ability to learn impacted your ability to succeed at life or your self-esteem? If yes, how so? Do you believe that your thinking can change? Do you believe that you have an incredibly powerful mind? Can you learn to be successfully *you*? Do you think that you can change the way you think, speak, and act and find meaning and purpose in your life?

_____

_____

_____

_____

_____

_____

# The Mindset Guide, Part 1

Read pages 35–72 in *Think, Learn, Succeed* and watch the key 2 video.

This section covers Thinking and Learning to Succeed, The Thinker Mindset, The Controlled Thinking Mindset, The Words Mindset, The Controlled Emotions Mindset, and The Forgiveness Mindset.

1. *A mindset is an attitude, or a cluster of thoughts with attached information and emotions that generate a particular perception.* What does the word *mindset* mean to you? How do mindsets impact our ability to think, learn, and succeed? Why is it important to have a good mindset?

_____

_____

_____

_____

_____

_____

_____

2. *Every moment of every day, your brain and body are physically reacting and changing in response to the thoughts that run through your mind—your mindsets add "flavor" to your thoughts, making your brain and body work for you or against you.* How do mindsets add "flavor" to your thoughts? Are mindsets powerful?

_____

_____

_____

_____

_____

_____

3. *The power of the mind to change the brain is incredibly exciting and hopeful!* How so? Have you seen this in your own life? How do you think you can use your mind to change your brain?

_____

_____

_____

_____

_____

4. *Think of your mind as the movement of information as energy through your nervous system.* How does this "movement" work? How can this "movement" be hijacked by negative thinking? How can we use this "movement" to our own advantage?

_____

_____

_____

_____

_____

_____

5. *Research in quantum physics and the mind-body connection shows the signals of the mind, which are considered nonphysical light waves or packets of energy, form 90 to 99 percent of who we are.* How so? Why is this important?

_____

_____

_____

_____

_____

6. *As long as you can breathe, your brain can make new neurons in a process called neurogenesis.* What is the importance of neurogenesis? How does it give us hope? How can we use neurogenesis to help us succeed in life?

_____

_____

_____

_____

7. *This process of reappraising and realigning your mindsets back to your natural wired-for-love design is integral to the life well-lived.* How do mindsets relate to changing the way we think? What is our "wired-for-love" design? Why is it important? How does it relate to our thinking?

_____

_____

_____

_____

_____

8. *Your thinking, feeling, and choosing impacts your genetic expression.* How so? Why is genetic expression important?

_____

_____

_____

_____

_____

_____

9. *We all think differently, which influences the effectiveness of building useful, sustainable memory.* What is the importance of thinking differently? How does recognizing the unique way we think, feel, and choose help us succeed?

_____

_____

_____

_____

_____

_____

10. *Your body and brain are finely attuned to your uniqueness and the positivity of your mind.* How so? How does this relate to our wired-for-love design? What happens when we step out of our wired-for-love design?

_____

_____

_____

_____

_____

_____

11. *Fear is distorted love.* What is "distorted love"? How does this impact our wired-for-love design? Can you think of examples of fear impacting your ability to function in your life?

_____

_____

_____

_____

_____

_____

12. *Brain plasticity means the changes that occur in the brain as a result of thinking and lifestyle choices.* What is "brain plasticity"? Why is it important? How can it help us succeed in life?

_____

_____

_____

_____

_____

13. *It is easy in today's age to have access to any number of readily accessible stimuli through social media, email, texting, ebooks, Facetime, Skype, chat rooms—you name it, you literally have a world of data at your fingertips.* How does this impact our ability to think and learn? How attached are you to technology? Do you think it has changed the way you think?

_____

_____

_____

_____

14. *You may be so connected that you have forgotten how to spend time just being alone with your thoughts.* Why is it important to be alone with your thoughts? Are you comfortable just "thinking"? If yes, why? If no, why? How do you "be alone with your thoughts"?

_____

_____

_____

_____

_____

_____

15. *Contrary to popular belief, the mind does not grind to a halt when you are doing nothing.* What happens when we just let our minds wander? Why is this an important part of mental self-care?

_____

_____

_____

_____

_____

16. *The mind-wandering "thinker" state can be highjacked, so to speak, by existing toxic thoughts moving up from our nonconscious mind, unless we control them.* How does this happen? Has this happened to you? How do we control these toxic thoughts?

_____

_____

_____

_____

_____

17. *We all face challenges in life, and we all need to learn how to consciously control our thought lives, every moment of every day, to cope and not break.* How have the challenges you have faced impacted your ability to cope with life? Do you think you can improve how you respond to the challenges of life? If yes, why? If no, why?

_____

_____

_____

_____

_____

_____

_____

_____

_____

_____

18. *Consciously controlling your thought life means that you do not allow thoughts to rampage through your mind.* How do you do this? Why is it important not to let thoughts "rampage through your mind"?

_____

_____

_____

_____

_____

_____

_____

_____

_____

19. *To control your thought life, you have to activate and continually make use of the quantum principle of* superposition, *which is the ability to focus on the incoming information and on upcoming memories from your nonconscious mind.* What is "superposition"? Why is it important? How can it help you control your thoughts? How does "superposition" relate to the Multiple Perspective Advantage (MPA)?

_____

_____

_____

_____

_____

_____

_____

_____

_____

_____

20. *When you use your mind to consciously take control of your thought life, you will find that it does not take long to see the benefits.* What are these benefits? Do you find that controlling your thinking improves the quality of your life? How so?

_____

_____

_____

_____

_____

_____

_____

_____

_____

_____

21. *The words you speak are electromagnetic and quantum life forces that come from thoughts inside your brain, which you build into your mind by thinking, feeling, and choosing over time.* What does this statement mean? How does this highlight the importance of what we say? How are words related to thoughts? Why are words powerful?

---

---

---

---

---

22. *Your words have to be backed up with honesty and integrity, or what in psychological terms is called cognitive congruence.* Why is it important to believe what you say? Why are positive affirmations alone not enough?

---

---

---

---

---

23. *Framing your world with your words, therefore, involves replacing negative thinking and words by changing your mindset.* How do we do this? What kind of words frame your world? Do you watch what you say?

---

---

---

---

---

24. *If you repress and hide toxic emotions, the time will come when those buried emotions will suddenly come pouring out.* Has this happened in your life? Do you hide your emotions?

_____

_____

_____

_____

_____

_____

25. *When you express your emotions in a healthy way, you allow the free flow of neuropeptides and energy, which allows all bodily systems to function as a healthy whole.* How so? What does it mean to express emotions in a "healthy way"? How do you do this? Why is it important?

_____

_____

_____

_____

_____

_____

26. *Acknowledging that you are expressing your uniquely created emotions in response to a particular situation is therefore an important step in detoxing your mind and brain.* Why is learning how to express your emotions important? How can you do this in your own life?

_____

_____

_____

_____

_____

_____

27. *We need to stop thinking we can interpret someone else's emotions.* Why is this a bad thing? Have you ever tried to figure out what someone is feeling without talking to them? If so, how did the situation turn out? Could you have handled it better?

_____

_____

_____

_____

_____

_____

28. *We're often told to "forgive and forget" the wrongs that we suffer, but it turns out that there is scientific truth (and gut logic) behind the common saying.* What happens when we forgive? Why is forgiveness important? How has forgiveness affected your own life?

_____

_____

_____

_____

_____

_____

29. *Adopting a forgiveness mindset is a choice, an act of your free will.* How is forgiveness a choice? How is it a mindset?

_____

_____

_____

_____

_____

30. *Forgiveness changes the brain.* How so? What happens to the brain if we do not forgive?

_____

_____

_____

_____

_____

_____

31. *It is not important how you forgive, just as long as you do—for your own sake as well as the sake of the people around you.* How does forgiveness help you? How does forgiveness help the people around you? Can you think of examples of forgiveness in your own life? What happens when you don't forgive someone?

_____

_____

_____

_____

_____

_____

32. *Forgiveness does not make excuses for someone's behavior.* What is the nature of forgiveness?

_____

_____

_____

_____

_____

KEY **3**

# The Mindset Guide, Part 2

> **Read pages 73–107 in** *Think, Learn,*
> *Succeed* **and watch the key 3 video.**

This section covers The Happiness Mindset, The Time Mindset, The Possible Mindset, The Gratitude Mindset, The Community Mindset, The Support Mindset, The Healthy Stress Mindset, The Expectancy Mindset, The Willpower Mindset, and The Spiritual Mindset.

1. *Happiness is a much wider and more nuanced concept than our capitalistic society would have us believe.* How do you define happiness? What do you think makes people happy? What are some of the ways our society defines happiness? What is a good way of defining happiness? Can happiness last, or is it fleeting?

_____

_____

_____

_____

_____

2. *Happiness precedes success.* What is the relationship between happiness and success? Do many people assume that they will be happy after they become successful? How do you view the relationship between success and happiness?

_____

_____

_____

_____

_____

_____

3. *Happiness does not mean a smooth and uncomplicated life.* How are happiness and challenges related? How do challenges help us live a successful and happy life? Do you feel like this is true in your life?

_____

_____

_____

_____

_____

_____

4. *Our happiness does not depend on our circumstances.* Is this true for your life? What does your happiness depend upon?

_____

_____

_____

_____

_____

_____

5. *Laughter and play are wonderful ways to reduce toxic stress and increase happiness.* How does having fun, laughing, and playing help us be happy? How does this help us succeed in life? How can you incorporate laughter and play into your life?

_____

_____

_____

_____

_____

_____

6. *Our goal for positive changes and success should last a lifetime.* What is the relationship between time and success? Is success instantaneous? Once we achieve success, do we rest on our laurels? Does the desire for success last a lifetime?

_____

_____

_____

_____

_____

_____

7. *We all know that change takes time and that there are challenges on the road to success, but few are willing to persevere.* Is this true in your life? Do you often find yourself giving up? What does perseverance look like? How does it relate to living a successful and happy life?

_____

_____

_____

_____

_____

_____

8. *We can turn dreams into realities, but we first have to realize that it takes longer than the average one-second lifespan of a Twitter post to make a change.* How has today's world changed the way we view success? What kind of expectations are associated with the speed of the technological revolution? Has the way we live today impacted your view or expectations of success?

_____

_____

_____

_____

_____

_____

_____

_____

_____

_____

9. *Like when you train your body to run a marathon or master a new exercise in the gym, your brain needs time to develop and achieve success, and you do this brain training with your mind.* How does the brain "train"? What kind of habits lead to a successful life? Does it take time to build these habits? Why?

_____

_____

_____

_____

_____

_____

_____

_____

_____

10. *An entrepreneurial focus sees multiple possibilities in every situation; it is a mindset that perceives all kinds of probabilities and potentialities.* Do you see multiple possibilities in situations? Or do you see only what is in front of you, as it is? If your plans do not work out, do you get thrown off? Why? What is an "entrepreneurial focus"? How does it lead to success?

_____

_____

_____

_____

_____

_____

_____

_____

_____

_____

11. *When you* choose *to develop a mindset that allows you to perceive possibilities, the wired-for-love design of the brain is activated to respond, and attempts become possibilities rather than failures.* How so? How can seeing possibilities be a choice?

_____

_____

_____

_____

_____

_____

_____

_____

_____

_____

12. *We cannot use our circumstances as an excuse not to succeed in life.* Have you ever used your circumstances as an excuse? What happens when we blame everyone and everything rather than taking responsibility for our own life?

_____

_____

_____

_____

_____

_____

13. *When we choose to be grateful, we tap into our natural design.* How so? What is our "natural design"? How does gratitude impact our success?

_____

_____

_____

_____

_____

_____

14. *An attitude of gratitude leads to the feeling that life is worth living, which brings mental health benefits in a positive feedback loop that leads to more resilience, the ability to bounce back more quickly.* How does gratitude relate to perseverance? How can gratitude affect our willpower? Have you experienced this in your own life?

_____

_____

_____

_____

_____

_____

15. *Human beings are social animals. Whether we like having alone time or not, we all need community.* Why is community important? What is the meaning of "social animal"? Do you feel the need to be part of a community in your own life? Why?

_____

_____

_____

_____

_____

16. *The more removed we become from human connection, the more potential there is for us to turn to the fantasy world as a replacement to reality, rather than using our imagination as a tool to create successful and satisfying lives.* Have you experienced this in your life? Why is isolation damaging to our health? How can isolation prevent us from succeeding in life?

_____

_____

_____

_____

_____

17. *We can all actively pursue a community mindset.* What is a "community mindset"? How can you pursue it? Why is this important?

_____

_____

_____

_____

_____

18. *High levels of social support predict longevity at least as reliably as healthy eating and regular exercise do, while low levels of social support are as damaging as high blood pressure.* What does this statement mean? Why is social support important? Do you have a good social support system in your life?

_____

_____

_____

_____

_____

_____

19. *Supportive relationships allow us to persevere through hard times.* How so? Is this true in your own life? What happens when we do not have a good social support system?

_____

_____

_____

_____

_____

_____

20. *Support is crucial in a learning environment.* Why? How does social support help us think, learn, and succeed in life?

_____

_____

_____

_____

_____

_____

21. *The way we view stressful situations can affect the way we deal with those situations.* How so? How can our perception of stress change the way stress affects us?

_____

_____

_____

_____

_____

_____

22. *When we read about the negative health effects of toxic stress, we certainly can get stressed-out about being stressed-out!* Has this happened to you? How do you think you can change the way you view stress?

_____

_____

_____

_____

_____

_____

23. *Due to the mind-body connection, expectancy produces real, neurophysiological outcomes in your body.* What is the "mind-body connection"? How do our expectations affect this connection? How have your expectations about a particular event or circumstance affected you? Do you expect things to go well? Why? Do you expect things to go badly? Why?

_____

_____

_____

_____

_____

_____

24. *Our expectations change the structure of our brains.* How so? How can you use your expectations to your advantage?

_____

_____

_____

_____

_____

_____

25. *Often, we have to push ourselves to do something we don't feel like doing.* Is this true in your own life? How do you push yourself to do something you don't want to do? What happens when you tap into your willpower?

_____

_____

_____

_____

_____

_____

26. *A willpower mindset is intimately connected to perseverance and is therefore directly linked to the expectancy mindset described above—it takes expectancy to the next level.* How does this happen? What is the importance of willpower? How does your attitude or perception of a situation affect your willpower? How can willpower change the way you think?

_____

_____

_____

_____

_____

_____

27. *For many people, spirituality is something that gives their lives purpose and shapes their thoughts, words, and actions.* Is this true in your life? How so? What is the relationship between spirituality, purpose, identity, and success?

_____

_____

_____

_____

_____

_____

28. *Spirituality is not a "delusion."* Why? How can spirituality be beneficial to our mental and physical health or our success?

_____

_____

_____

_____

_____

_____

29. *Each of us has our own unique "flavor," our own unique way of thinking, feeling, and choosing, and this is reflected through our mindsets.* What does this statement mean? What is the relationship between our unique way of thinking and our mindsets? Why is this relationship important?

_____

_____

_____

_____

_____

_____

KEY **4**

# The Gift Profile, Part 1

> **Read pages 109–48 in** *Think, Learn,*
> *Succeed* **and watch the key 4 video.**

1. *We each have an exclusive blueprint of thinking, a way of thinking that needs to be designed by us for us.* What is our "blueprint of thinking"? Why is it important? Do you think that everyone thinks in a customized way?

_____

_____

_____

_____

2. *As we think, we create these customized exclusive realities.* What does this statement mean? Have you observed this in your own life?

_____

_____

_____

_____

3. *Thinking is a process and goes through a cycle, just like digestion.* How so? What is the importance of this cycle?

_____

_____

_____

_____

_____

_____

4. *Our customized way of thinking is the unique way each of our minds in action moves through the brain.* What is the "mind in action"? How does it operate through the brain? Is this process different for each of us?

_____

_____

_____

_____

_____

_____

5. *We need to learn to capitalize on how our customized thinking works in our brains so that we can function at the highest level possible to achieve success in life.* How does understanding the unique way we think help us succeed? Has this happened in your life?

_____

_____

_____

_____

_____

_____

6. *No two individuals are alike.* How are we all different?

_____

_____

_____

_____

_____

_____

_____

_____

7. *Changing the activity of the mind can alter the way basic genetic instructions are implemented.* How does thinking affect genetic expression? Why is this important?

_____

_____

_____

_____

_____

_____

_____

8. *We all have different opinions; we all think differently; we all speak and act differently.* Why do you think it is important to understand how we think and how other people think?

_____

_____

_____

_____

_____

_____

9. *Understanding your customized mode of thinking, how you digest information, helps you understand how your mind works, thus activating correct mindsets.* How so? How does customized thinking relate to the correct mindsets?

_____

_____

_____

_____

_____

_____

10. *The mind is separate from the brain. The mind works through the substrate of the brain, which, in turn, responds to the mind.* What does this statement mean? How can the mind be different from the brain? How is this different from neuroreductionism?

_____

_____

_____

_____

_____

_____

11. *We need to exercise caution when we read studies or articles on the brain.* Why? How can the misinterpretation of brain studies be dangerous?

_____

_____

_____

_____

_____

12. *As science progresses, researchers are getting glimpses into the minute intricate structures of the brain that highlight the brain's complex quantum nature.* What is this "complex quantum nature"? Why is it important? How is it changing the way we view thinking and the brain?

_____

_____

_____

_____

_____

_____

13. *Essentially, every thought you have is a complex piece of music you have written with your choices, a piece that plays out in your brain and in your life.* What does this statement mean? Have you observed this in your own life? Why is this important?

_____

_____

_____

_____

_____

_____

14. *The brain is a complex machine. In addition to the two hemispheres, four lobes, and numerous structures of the brain, there is an additional theorized arrangement of seven modules that run from top to bottom and left to right across the brain.* What are these seven modules? Why are they important?

_____

_____

_____

_____

_____

15. *The Gift Profile I developed over twenty years ago and have expanded over the last ten years is a way of gaining insight into the mysterious world of thinking.* What is the Gift Profile? What does it tell us about ourselves? How does it work?

_____

_____

_____

_____

_____

_____

16. *Each metacognitive module has a general umbrella-type function.* What does this statement mean? What are the different functions of the seven modules of thought?

_____

_____

_____

_____

_____

_____

17. *As you think in your own customized way, your brain kicks into high gear and you operate like a fine-tuned car with all seven types of thought oiled into thinking "it" through.* How so? Why is this process important? Is this process the same for all of us? Do these modules operate in isolation?

_____

_____

_____

_____

_____

_____

18. *When it comes to filling in any type of profile, we always need to bear in mind that there is no single profile assessment or test that can define the complexity of humanity.* Does the Gift Profile tell you everything you need to know about your thinking? Or is it a "blueprint" that allows you to begin discovering your unique way of thinking?

_____

_____

_____

_____

_____

19. *Research shows that intelligence is unique to each of us. Talent is not fixed; it grows and develops with us as we use it.* Why is this significant? How do you view intelligence?

_____

_____

_____

_____

_____

20. *It is important to remember that although our thought-life is a "stream of consciousness," with thousands of individual thoughts blending together, we can control what we allow into our heads.* Do you feel like you can control what you think? If yes, how? If no, why?

_____

_____

_____

_____

_____

21. *In terms of the cycle of thought, you will only really be aware of the first two types of thought among the seven modules, and perhaps your last two in your order. Why? Is thinking a slow or fast process?*

_____

_____

_____

_____

_____

_____

Before you continue on to the next section,
complete the Gift Profile.

# The Gift Profile, Part 2

Read pages 149–69 in *Think, Learn,*
*Succeed* **and watch the key 5 video.**

1. *Intrapersonal thinking is, at its heart, the ability to stand outside of ourselves and analyze our own thinking.* What is intrapersonal thinking? What does this look like in your own life?

_____

_____

_____

_____

_____

2. *You are introspective and aware of your range of emotions.* What module of thinking is this? What are the other characteristics of this module of thinking? How can you develop this type of thinking?

_____

_____

_____

_____

_____

3. *Interpersonal thinking gives us the ability to understand and work with people.* How so? What does this look like in your own life?

_____

_____

_____

_____

_____

_____

4. *You love to talk.* What module of thinking is this? What are the other characteristics of this module of thinking? How can you develop this type of thinking?

_____

_____

_____

_____

_____

_____

5. *The Linguistic module of thinking deals with how you use language to express yourself.* What does this mean? What does this look like in your own life?

_____

_____

_____

_____

_____

_____

_____

6. *Semantics is the meanings or connotation of words.* Can you think of an example of semantics? What are the other domains of language?

_____

_____

_____

_____

_____

_____

7. *You like to write, play with words, read, and tell stories.* What module of thinking is this? What are the other characteristics of this module of thinking? How can you develop this type of thinking?

_____

_____

_____

_____

_____

_____

8. *The Logical/Mathematical module of thinking deals with scientific reasoning, logic, and analysis.* What is Logical/Mathematical thinking? What does this look like in your own life?

_____

_____

_____

_____

_____

_____

9. *Pattern recognition is the ability to categorize, organize, and make associations in nature, numbers, words, stories, and life.* Can you think of an example of pattern recognition? What are the other domains of logic and mathematics?

_____

_____

_____

_____

_____

_____

10. *You love to roam in the realm of imaginary and irrational numbers.* What module of thinking is this? What are the other characteristics of this module of thinking? How can you develop this type of thinking?

_____

_____

_____

_____

_____

11. *The Kinesthetic module of thinking includes movement, somatic sensation, and moving around.* What does this look like in your own life? Can you think of some examples of this type of thinking?

_____

_____

_____

_____

_____

_____

12. *You explore your environment through touch and movement.* What module of thinking is this? What are the other characteristics of this module of thinking? How can you develop this type of thinking?

_____

_____

_____

_____

_____

_____

13. *The Musical module of thinking helps you to develop your instinct, allowing you to read between the lines in various situations.* Does Musical thinking just involve music? What is Musical thinking? What does this look like in your own life?

_____

_____

_____

_____

_____

_____

14. *You instinctively feel when things are right or wrong.* What module of thinking is this? What are the other characteristics of this module of thinking? How can you develop this type of thinking?

_____

_____

_____

_____

_____

_____

15. *The Visual/Spatial module of thinking deals with the ability to see color, light, shape, and depth.* What is Visual/Spatial thinking? What does this look like in your own life?

_____

_____

_____

_____

_____

_____

16. *You enjoy hands-on activities. That is, you learn by seeing and doing.* What module of thinking is this? What are the other characteristics of this module of thinking? How can you develop this type of thinking?

_____

_____

_____

_____

_____

_____

17. *As you analyze your profile, remember that you cannot be put in a box. If Logical/Mathematical happens to be at the bottom of the order of your gifts, and you aren't that great at math, it doesn't matter.* Why doesn't it matter? Can you develop your gifting? How does this development affect all the thinking modules?

_____

_____

_____

_____

_____

_____

18. *Using your customized thinking can be tremendously rewarding.* How do you think that it will benefit you?

_____

_____

_____

_____

_____

_____

_____

19. *Your customized way of thinking operates a bit like dominoes.* How so?

_____

_____

_____

_____

_____

_____

20. *Essentially, there are an infinite number of thinking patterns, each giving rise to another thinking pattern or gift.* What does this mean for the way we think, speak, and act? How does this realization change the way we see and develop our thinking? Can we label people?

_____

_____

_____

_____

_____

_____

21. *When you continually use your customized thinking, you can enhance and preserve the brain's powers as you move through life.* How so? How is this beneficial as we age?

_____

_____

_____

_____

_____

_____

22. *The gift concept helps us to see each other as different and unique. We understand that our differences are not a threat.* How does this help us not feel threatened by others? Can we compare ourselves to anyone? How does this relate to the notion of community?

_____

_____

_____

_____

_____

_____

23. *We need to focus on what we can do, rather than what we think we can't do.* How does understanding our customized thinking help us to do this? How can this change the way we educate people?

_____

_____

_____

_____

_____

24. *Each one of us is a special part of this wonderfully unique puzzle that is life.* How does our customized way of thinking tie into our purpose?

_____

_____

_____

_____

_____

_____

25. *If the brain is the physical substrate through which the mind works, the place where our thoughts are stored and from which we speak and act, then each human brain is uniquely attuned to each person.* Why do we think differently? And why is this important?

_____

_____

_____

_____

_____

_____

26. *Our views of the world are reflected in the architecture of our brains.* What does this statement mean? How is it related to our customized way of thinking?

_____

_____

_____

_____

_____

# The Switch On Your Brain 5-Step Learning Process, Part 1

> Read pages 171–80 in *Think, Learn, Succeed* and watch the key 6 video.

1. *Mindfulness is the ability to bring attention to our self-awareness, to recognize how we are thinking or feeling at any one moment.* Why is mindfulness important? How do you understand mindfulness?

_____

_____

_____

_____

_____

_____

_____

_____

_____

_____

_____

2. *Going* beyond *mindfulness means that you redirect the calm, organized, and insightful state gained from mindfulness into an extremely productive knowledge-gaining process, a process that enhances and cultivates the information you receive in a successful way for whatever purpose you need it.* What does "going beyond mindfulness" mean? Why is this important? How does it help us succeed in life?

_____

_____

_____

_____

_____

3. *Learning how to learn and build sustainable memory will not only get you where you want to go but also improve your mental and physical health.* How so? Why is learning how to learn so important? How does this relate to going "beyond mindfulness"?

_____

_____

_____

_____

4. *The technological revolution, notwithstanding its many benefits, has also impacted the way we think.* How so? Can you think of some examples of this in your life? Why is it so important that we learn how to learn since the technological revolution?

_____

_____

_____

_____

_____

5. *An overreliance on computers and search engines is weakening people's focus, deep thinking, attention, and memory.* How so? Do you find that this is true in your own life?

_____

_____

_____

_____

_____

6. *We have to start at mindfulness but go beyond it to create new meaningful habituated memories, or we won't create sustainable and maintainable change in our lives.* What does this statement mean? What is "sustainable" change? How can we develop a habit or pattern of deep and focused learning in our lives?

_____

_____

_____

_____

_____

7. *We need to make digital technology platforms work for us and not against us.* How can we do this? Can you think of ways of making technology work for you in your life?

_____

_____

_____

_____

_____

8. *Healthy, productive learning is good, old-fashioned hard work that draws on the amazing capacity we have as humans to think and learn—the opposite of what the incorrect use of technology does.* What is learning? How do you learn? Do you learn with understanding? Is learning a quick process?

_____

_____

_____

_____

_____

9. *We shouldn't be tempted to fall for the gadgets, gizmos, tricks, or DIY guides that promise to make us smarter and more intelligent overnight.* Have you ever found yourself doing this? What happened? Can you think of some examples of learning "tricks" or "gizmos" that promise instant success?

_____

_____

_____

_____

_____

10. *Research indicates that as we grow more dependent on technology, so intellect weakens and addictions rise.* What is this research? Why is it important? How can bad learning affect our mental and physical health? Have you found this to be true in your own life?

_____

_____

_____

_____

_____

11. *Mental self-care incorporates understanding and using the power of mindsets by activating our customized thinking, which, in turn, allows us to build the brain through learning to build useful memory.* How does learning relate to mindsets and customized thinking? Why is this "mental self-care"?

_____

_____

_____

_____

_____

_____

_____

12. *We need to take responsibility for thinking and learning to succeed.* Why is learning a responsibility?

_____

_____

_____

_____

_____

_____

13. *Thoughts occupy mental real estate.* What does this statement mean? How does it relate to learning?

_____

_____

_____

_____

_____

_____

14. *The physical representation of thoughts in the brain looks like trees but are actual clusters of neurons with dendrites.* What are dendrites? Why are they important?

_____

_____

_____

_____

_____

_____

_____

15. *Learning builds memories, and memories are used to express our mindsets, worldview, and, most importantly, our "youness."* Why is your customized way of thinking important when it comes to learning?

_____

_____

_____

_____

_____

_____

_____

16. *Whatever you think about the most grows in your mind.* Why is it important to watch what you are learning?

_____

_____

_____

_____

_____

_____

_____

17. *Your mind can rebuild and restrengthen your memory, even when your brain has gone through the traumas of life.* Do you feel like this is true in your life? Is learning possible if you have been through physical and mental trauma? Can the brain heal?

_____

_____

_____

_____

_____

_____

_____

_____

_____

_____

18. *My initial research focused on traumatic brain injury (TBI) and on people with learning disabilities, autism, chronic traumatic encephalopathy (CTE), and cerebral palsy, as well as those suffering from cognitive, communicative, and emotional pathologies and dementias.* What was my original research? What did it show?

_____

_____

_____

_____

_____

_____

_____

_____

_____

# The Switch On Your Brain 5-Step Learning Process, Part 2

Read pages 180–204 in *Think, Learn, Succeed* and watch the key 7 video.

1. *The Switch On Your Brain 5-Step Learning Process is made up of five important steps that facilitate this disciplined and directed learning process I discuss in my book* Think, Learn, Succeed. What are these five steps? Why are they important? How do they help with the learning process?

_____

_____

_____

_____

_____

_____

_____

_____

_____

2. *The easy-come, easy-go neuronal connections that come from lack of deep processing, rote learning, cramming for exams or meetings, and relying on digital platforms are quickly reversed.* What does this mean? How does this type of learning affect the brain? Have you found this to be true in your own life? How is the five-step learning process different?

_____

_____

_____

_____

_____

3. *Your thinking can change the structure of your brain, which is called* mind-directed *neuroplasticity.* What is the significance of "*mind-directed* neuroplasticity"? How does it relate to learning and mental self-care?

_____

_____

_____

_____

_____

4. *The entorhinal cortex is responsible for the preprocessing of input signals (the information) and is an important memory center in the brain.* What is the entorhinal cortex? How is it an important "memory center"?

_____

_____

_____

_____

_____

5. *You need to see* and hear *the words you are reading.* What does this statement mean? How does it relate to inputting information? What are the other ways we make sure that we are inputting information into the brain correctly?

_____

_____

_____

_____

_____

6. *As you input information into the brain by listening and reading and experiencing through your five senses, the information passes through the brain on two levels.* What are these two levels? How does this process of inputting or entering information in the brain work? Why is it important?

_____

_____

_____

_____

_____

7. *The Golden Rule of the Switch On Your Brain 5-Step Learning Process is to* think to understand *the information you are trying to remember.* What does it mean to understand what you are "trying to remember"? What are the three steps that help you "think to understand"?

_____

_____

_____

_____

_____

8. *Stop and* ask *yourself what you have just read.* How does this relate to the Focused Thinking step? Why is this important? What are the other ways you can focus your thinking?

_____

_____

_____

_____

_____

_____

9. *The Focused Thinking step challenges the brain to move into a higher gear, which is what it is designed for: deep, intellectual thought!* How does the brain move into a higher gear? Why is this important? What is deep, intellectual thought?

_____

_____

_____

_____

_____

_____

10. *This way of writing down information [Metacogs] looks like the branching of dendrites on neurons.* What are Metacogs? How do they reflect the structure of the brain? Why are they important? How do they work?

_____

_____

_____

_____

_____

_____

11. *You naturally and instinctively try to work out its meaning, which is the essential 15 to 35 percent of concepts per sentence.* How does this process relate to building a Metacog? How do you build a Metacog?

_____

_____

_____

_____

_____

_____

12. *As you use a Metacog, the frontal lobe, parietal lobe, temporal lobe, and occipital lobe of your brain all work together to integrate and apply the information.* How does this happen? Why is this important?

_____

_____

_____

_____

_____

_____

13. *Recheck/Revisit is a very simple yet extremely powerful process.* What is this process? Why is it powerful? How do you recheck or revisit information?

_____

_____

_____

_____

_____

_____

14. *The Recheck/Revisit stage allows you to consolidate and re-inforce memory of your work*. How so? How do you recheck your information?

_____

_____

_____

_____

_____

_____

_____

15. *In the Output/Reteach step, you need to play "teacher" and sequentially reteach all the information that is on your Metacog.* Why is this important? How can you do this?

_____

_____

_____

_____

_____

_____

_____

16. *The Output/Reteach step also creates new connections*. What do these new connections look like in the brain?

_____

_____

_____

_____

_____

_____

_____

17. *Today, more than ever before, there are no limits to what you can achieve, especially when equipped with the right tools.* Do you believe this statement? If yes, why? If no, why? Why are there "no limits" to what you can achieve?

_____

_____

_____

_____

_____

_____

_____

_____

18. *The five steps, with the third-step Metacog, are also a great note-taking tool in meetings and lectures.* What are some of the other ways you can use Metacogs? How can the Metacog be a useful tool in your life?

_____

_____

_____

_____

_____

_____

_____

_____

**Practice using the Switch On Your Brain 5-Step Learning Process before you continue on to the next section. Use it with any type of information that interests you, or use it to learn a new skill or study for a test/exam/review.**

# The Science, Part 1

Read pages 205–26 in *Think, Learn,*
*Succeed* and watch the key 8 video.

1. *We experience events all the time, all day long. We are also react-*
   *ing to these events all day long.* What does this statement mean?
   How do we react to events? What are these reactions called? What
   is the "mind-in-action"? Why is it important?

   _____

   _____

   _____

   _____

   _____

2. *We forget certain things because we need to for brain health.* How
   is forgetting related to our mental and physical health? Do you
   find that this is true in your own life?

   _____

   _____

   _____

   _____

3. *Many people are misdiagnosed and labeled and put in a box when there wasn't a box to begin with.* Can you think of some examples of these labels? Why are they bad? Have you ever been labeled? How did this label change the way you perceived yourself and your abilities? What effect did it have on your life?

_____

_____

_____

_____

_____

4. *For many years, the prevailing wisdom was that memory was stored in the synaptic connections between neurons.* What does this statement mean? How has our view of memory changed? Why has it changed?

_____

_____

_____

_____

_____

5. *We all want to build the kind of memory that will lead to success. To do so, we need to* think *in such a way that will engage our dendrites to build memory that leads to success in the* long run. What kind of memory is important for success? How do we build this memory? How do we make sure we build strong memories that last?

_____

_____

_____

_____

_____

_____

6. *Synaptic connections are a bit like meeting someone for the first time.* What does this statement mean? What are synaptic connections?

_____

_____

_____

_____

_____

_____

_____

7. *Your thinking is phenomenally fast—every thought you think impacts every single one of the 75 to 100 trillion cells of your body in an instant.* Why is the thinking process so fast?

_____

_____

_____

_____

_____

_____

8. *Each thought we think is in fact a veritable universe.* What does this statement mean regarding our potential to succeed at life? Do you find that each of your own thoughts is a "veritable universe"? If yes, why? If no, why?

_____

_____

_____

_____

_____

9. *Dendrites, working with synapses and cell bodies through quantum action, appear designed to do the job of thinking.* How so? What are dendrites?

_____

_____

_____

_____

_____

_____

10. *The brain, as a quantum computer, can calculate different computations simultaneously in response to the mind-in-action process of decision making.* How so? What are "quantum rain clouds"? Why are they important? How do they relate to free will and our ability to choose?

_____

_____

_____

_____

_____

_____

11. *If we go inside the neurons, we find an incredible wonderland: miniscule little tubes called microtubules, around ten million per neuron.* What are microtubules? Why are they important? What is their relationship to short-term memory?

_____

_____

_____

_____

_____

_____

12. *The more we think in our own customized way, the more coherence we will have, enabling us to make positive choices when we are in superposition.* What does this statement mean? Why is our customized way of thinking important for memory formation? What is "superposition"? Why is it important? What is Heisenberg's uncertainty principle? Why is it important?

_____

_____

_____

_____

_____

13. *This collapse of the wave function (or cloud) is also called de-coherence in quantum theory.* What does this statement mean? Why is decoherence important?

_____

_____

_____

_____

_____

14. *For successful and useful memory to start forming, we need to choose to deliberately and intentionally regulate our thinking through focusing and paying attention to what we allow into our heads.* How do we do this? What is the Quantum Zeno Effect, and why is it an important part of memory formation?

_____

_____

_____

_____

_____

15. *Successful long-term memory requires more time and more work.* What does this statement mean? How is long-term memory different from short-term memory?

_____

_____

_____

_____

_____

_____

16. *The more you practice deliberate, self-regulatory thinking by using the techniques in this book, the more your brain will respond—you are literally redesigning your brain as you think!* What is "deliberate, self-regulatory thinking"? How can you redesign your brain with your thoughts?

_____

_____

_____

_____

_____

_____

17. *There are three levels of thinking.* What are these three levels of thinking? Why are they important? How do they relate to the Switch On Your Brain 5-Step Learning Process?

_____

_____

_____

_____

_____

_____

18. *A memory is only useful if you automatize it.* What does this statement mean?

_____

_____

_____

_____

_____

_____

_____

19. *Unfortunately, most people give up within the first week of learning and do not push through.* Is this true in your own life? If yes, why? If no, why?

_____

_____

_____

_____

_____

_____

_____

20. *"Snowflakes" are subsequently transformed into a six-legged shape that is fondly called a Nano Poodle.* What does this statement mean? What are these "snowflakes"? What are "Nano Poodles," and what part do they play in memory formation?

_____

_____

_____

_____

_____

_____

_____

21. *Tubulins have another really interesting characteristic: they self-assemble and reassemble.* What does this statement mean? What are tubulins? Why are they important?

_____

_____

_____

_____

_____

_____

_____

22. *The brain responds to the mind. Quantum theory is a way of understanding this interaction between the mind and the brain; it uses mathematics to describe this relationship.* How does quantum theory help us understand how the brain responds to the mind?

_____

_____

_____

_____

_____

_____

_____

23. *We have a lot of control over what goes on inside our heads. We are not merely dancing to the tune of our atoms or our DNA.* How so? How does this statement relate to quantum theory?

_____

_____

_____

_____

_____

24. *Quantum physics helps us understand just how entangled and dependent our world is.* What is entanglement in quantum physics? Why is it important?

_____

_____

_____

_____

_____

_____

# The Science, Part 2

> Read pages 227–40 in *Think, Learn, Succeed* and watch the key 9 video.

1. *The Geodesic Information Processing Theory is the theory that I first developed nearly thirty years ago and have updated in the intervening years.* What is my theory? Why is it important? How are the tools in this book based on my theory?

   _____

   _____

   _____

   _____

   _____

2. *There are seven metacognitive modules.* Can you remember what these modules are, and why they are important? Do they work together?

   _____

   _____

   _____

   _____

3. *Each metacognitive module has four processing systems.* What are the four processing systems?

_____

_____

_____

_____

_____

_____

_____

4. *Each processing system is broken down into three metacognitive domains.* What are these domains?

_____

_____

_____

_____

_____

_____

5. *These metacognitive domains provide the structure of the* descriptive systems *(memories).* What does this statement mean? What are "descriptive memories"?

_____

_____

_____

_____

_____

_____

_____

6. *The activity happening in these components is controlled by mind-in-action regulation—your thinking, feeling, and choosing.* What is mind-in-action regulation? What is the difference between dynamic self-regulation and active self-regulation?

_____

_____

_____

_____

_____

_____

7. Metacognitive action *is the term for the deep thinking that causes the what, how, and when/why elements of your memory to start interacting through deliberate, intentional thinking.* How does metacognitive action relate to mind-in-action regulation?

_____

_____

_____

_____

_____

_____

8. *These seven modules are not exhaustive but rather representative of the broad range of human knowledge and intellectual potential.* How so? How are they different for each person? How do they work in an entangled way?

_____

_____

_____

_____

_____

_____

9. *The seven metacognitive modules of my theory differ from the seven intelligences of Howard Gardner's "multiple intelligences" theory.* How are they different?

_____

_____

_____

_____

_____

_____

10. *A processing system is represented neurologically as a functional structure composed of interrelations of different parts of the brain.* How do processing systems work in the brain? How does this relate to our gift, or our customized way of thinking?

_____

_____

_____

_____

_____

_____

_____

11. *In order to be able to read that book or give that speech, you need to activate or operationalize the processing system.* What is this activation called?

_____

_____

_____

_____

_____

_____

12. *Your nonconscious mind does not stop analyzing, cleaning up, reading, and integrating all the memories you have, which are changing and growing in response to the experiences of your daily life.* How is this different from the conscious mind?

_____

_____

_____

_____

_____

13. *Dynamic self-regulation controls up to 90 percent of thinking and learning. It is responsible for activating and energizing long-term memories and belief systems (worldviews) to move into our conscious awareness and, as such, has an enormous influence on our conscious thinking, feeling, and choosing.* What does this statement mean? Why is this so important?

_____

_____

_____

_____

_____

14. *Active self-regulation is intentional and controlled by your choice to pay attention to something. Its effectiveness is determined by how mindful and deliberate you are in any given moment.* What does this statement mean? How does this interact with dynamic self-regulation? How is it different from dynamic self-regulation?

_____

_____

_____

_____

_____

15. *Metacognitive domains use declarative (what), procedural (how), and conditional (when/why) types of knowledge to build pattern-nature memories (descriptive systems).* What does this statement mean?

_____

_____

_____

_____

_____

_____

16. *Every moment of every day we are merging with our environment.* How so? Why is this important? Why should we be aware of our environment?

_____

_____

_____

_____

_____

_____

17. *The particular way you build and store memories is based on your specific perceptions and interpretations, which are exclusive to you.* How does this relate to our customized way of thinking?

_____

_____

_____

_____

_____

_____

18. *When a particular form of information is presented, your mind goes into action and works through the substrate of your brain.* How so?

_____

_____

_____

_____

_____

_____

19. *Deep thinking is called* metacognitive action, *which is when the what, how, and when/why elements of your memory start interacting through deliberate thinking until they generate enough energy to move into your conscious mind.* How so? Why is deep thinking important? What does deep, mindful thinking look like in the brain?

_____

_____

_____

_____

_____

20. *Metacognitive action is your deep thinking, feeling, and choosing, expressed as the fundamental elements of the way you think.* How do you understand metacognitive action? How does it relate to "readiness potential"?

_____

_____

_____

_____

_____

_____

21. *Benjamin Libet, a pioneer in the field of human consciousness, performed one of the first studies on cognition and metacognition.* What was this study? Why is it important?

_____

_____

_____

_____

_____

_____

22. *The brain, as a physical substrate, appears to be responding to (or is being "used" by) the nonconscious mind, which is orchestrated by dynamic self-regulation and the process of selecting the appropriate descriptive systems (memories) that need to move to the conscious mind.* How does this relate to free will?

_____

_____

_____

_____

_____

23. *The difference between your customized thinking and mine appears to involve differences in the components of the seven metacognitive modules, their metacognitive domains, and their processing systems.* How so?

_____

_____

_____

_____

_____

_____

24. *When we move out of our customized thinking, we do not tap into the modules correctly.* What happens in our brain and body when we move out of our customized way of thinking? Have you observed this in your own life?

_____

_____

_____

_____

_____

_____

_____

25. *Learning is the creative reconceptualization of knowledge.* What does this statement mean? What is the purpose of learning? Is this true in your own life?

_____

_____

_____

_____

_____

_____

_____

26. *Whatever we focus on the most will grow and influence our perspectives and belief systems (or worldviews).* How does this relate to learning? Why is this important?

_____

_____

_____

_____

_____

_____

# Conclusion

Congratulations, you have completed the *Think, Learn, Succeed Workbook*! You are on your way to using the incredible power that is in your mind to learn and succeed in every area of your life.

Remember, mindsets contain power, customized thinking activates this power, and the five-step process builds this power into long-term sustainable change. This a *lifestyle* of mental self-care. Do not fall for quick tricks, fancy gadgets, or neuromyths. There is no simple or quick program that will give you purpose or help you succeed in life. It takes good, old-fashioned hard work and a habit of deep, intentional thinking to get ahead in school, the workplace, or life. Fundamentally, *how you understand and use your mind is predictive of how successful you will be.*

Never fall into the trap of comparing your life to someone else's and thinking you are "not doing something right." We all think, feel, and choose in unique ways; we all define our own meaningful success. The book, workbook, and DVD are all about helping you get to that place to succeed, to make that switch to a life well-lived, filled with *meaningful* success, not the kind of success that is here for a moment and gone the next. Success is not about how many cars you have or what your house looks like or what your job title is or how sexy your beach body is, even though these things can be nice. Success is about being the best version of yourself you can be, regardless of your circumstances. It is about being proud of what you see in the mirror and the kind of impact you have on the people around you.

Success is about being you, as only you can be. Remember, you are as successful as *you* want to be.

**Dr. Caroline Leaf** is the author of *Switch On Your Brain*, *Think and Eat Yourself Smart*, and *The Perfect You*, among many other books and journal articles. Since 1981, she has researched the science of thought and the mind-brain connection as it relates to thinking, learning, renewing the mind, gifting, and potential. Dr. Leaf practiced clinically for twenty-five years and is an international and national conference speaker on topics relating to optimal brain performance such as learning, mindful thinking, stress, toxic thoughts, male/female brain differences, mindful eating, and much more. She is frequently interviewed on TV stations around the globe, has published many books and scientific journal articles, and has her own TV show, *The Dr. Leaf Show*. She and her husband, Mac, live with their four children in Dallas and Los Angeles.